# Master the Inverted Row for Maximum Core Activation

# A Bodyweight Ab Workout

## Helen Talbott

# Disclaimer

This book, (Master the Inverted Row for Maximum Core Activation), is intended for informational purposes only and should not be construed as medical advice. The information presented within is based on the author's research and experience, but individual circumstances and needs may vary.

Always consult with a qualified healthcare professional before incorporating any new exercise program or making changes to your existing routine, especially if you have any pre-existing conditions or injuries.

The author and publisher expressly disclaim any responsibility or liability for any injuries or health problems arising from the use of the information contained within this book.

Specific Disclaimers:

- While the inverted row exercise is presented as a beneficial exercise, it is crucial to practice proper form and technique to avoid injury. This book strives to provide clear instructions and illustrations, but ultimately, the responsibility for safe execution lies with the reader.
- The information on nutrition and supplementation included in this book is for general guidance only and is not intended to diagnose, treat, or cure any medical condition. Readers should consult with a registered dietitian or other qualified healthcare professional for personalized dietary advice.
- The use of specific workout programs, variations, or progressions suggested in this book is at the reader's own risk. Always listen to your body, modify exercises as needed, and discontinue if you experience any pain or discomfort.
- Any external links or resources mentioned in this book are provided for informational

purposes only and do not constitute an endorsement by the author or publisher. Readers should exercise their own judgment when accessing and using any external information.

By choosing to engage in the exercises and activities described in this book, you acknowledge and accept these disclaimers and release the author and publisher from any and all liability.

Remember, your health and safety are paramount. Consult with a healthcare professional before starting any new exercise program or making significant changes to your lifestyle.

**Table of contents**

# About the author

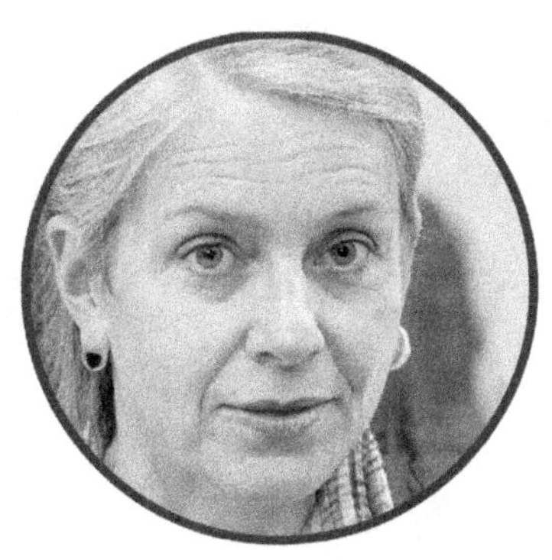

Helen Talbott is not just a name on the cover; it's a testament to a lifelong passion for movement and its transformative potential. As a certified personal trainer and fitness enthusiast, Helen's journey began with a personal quest for strength and empowerment. But soon, her passion took shape, guiding her to share the transformative power of movement with others.

Through insightful writing and accessible language, Helen paints a vivid picture of the human body's potential, using the inverted row as a powerful metaphor for inner strength and personal growth. Her approach is rooted in science-backed knowledge, yet infused with empathy and a genuine understanding of the challenges and triumphs that come with any fitness journey.

So, delve into the world of Helen Talbott, and uncover not just a writer or a trainer, but a passionate advocate for self-discovery and empowerment through movement. Remember, the strength you seek isn't just in your muscles; it lies within, waiting to be unlocked. Let Helen guide you on that journey.

The inverted row used to be my nemesis. Seeing those gym rats effortlessly pull themselves up with their bodies parallel to the ground filled me with envy and self-doubt. "There's no way I can do that," I'd mutter, feeling my skinny arms protest at the mere thought. But something within me yearned for that strength, that feeling of defying gravity.

Fueled by this desire, I decided to conquer my fear. Starting with pathetic attempts using resistance bands, I diligently practiced, focusing on form and pushing myself bit by bit. The initial frustration was intense, but each successful rep became a victory, a testament to my growing strength.

The journey wasn't smooth. There were days when my grip failed, my core gave out, and self-doubt crept in. But each setback became a stepping stone.

Slowly but surely, I started seeing results. My body grew stronger, my posture improved, and my confidence soared. The once impossible exercise became a source of empowerment. I wasn't just pulling myself up; I was pulling myself beyond my limitations.

Today, the inverted row is no longer a nemesis but a trusted friend. It's a reminder of how far I've come, of the strength I never knew I possessed.

# Introduction

Why the Inverted Row is the Ultimate Core Exercise

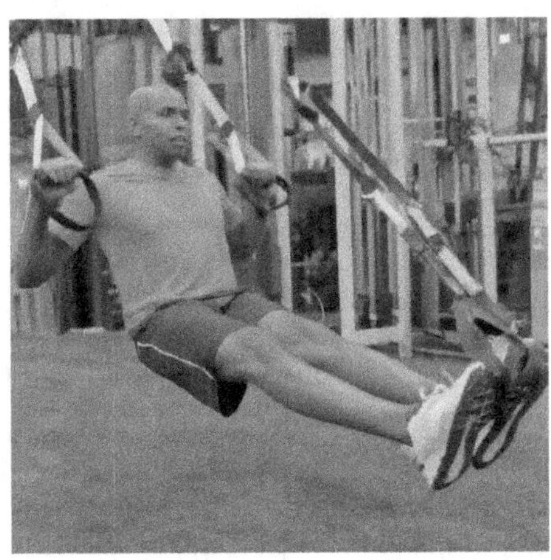

Forget endless crunches and sit-ups! Are you ready to unlock a hidden gem for building a strong, powerful, and defined core? Look no further than the inverted row. This seemingly simple exercise, often overlooked or misused, holds the key to unleashing your core potential and sculpting the abs you've always dreamed of.

But why is the inverted row so special for your core? Here's the truth:

1. More than just abs: It's true, the inverted row directly targets your abs, engaging them throughout the entire movement. But it doesn't stop there. This exercise simultaneously challenges your back muscles, shoulders, and even your grip, creating a synergistic effect that builds functional core strength, the kind that translates to real-world activities and improved athletic performance.

2. Anti-rotation powerhouse: Forget isolated crunches that only train one plane of motion. The inverted row forces your core to resist rotational forces, mimicking real-life movements and building anti-rotational strength. This is crucial for protecting your

spine from injury and improving stability in all your activities.

3. Scalable for all levels: Don't be intimidated if you can't pull yourself up yet. The inverted row is incredibly versatile and can be modified to suit any fitness level. Whether you're a beginner using an assisted machine or an advanced athlete performing weighted variations, the inverted row provides a scalable challenge that keeps you progressing.

4. Bodyweight advantage: No fancy equipment needed! The inverted row utilizes your own bodyweight as resistance, making it an accessible and efficient exercise for anyone, anywhere.

5. Functional core, sculpted abs: By building a strong and functional core with the inverted row, you'll naturally develop a defined and toned abdominal region. Think beyond the

"six-pack" and embrace a core that's both aesthetically pleasing and incredibly powerful.

In this guide, we'll delve deeper into why the inverted row deserves the title of "ultimate core exercise." We'll explore the anatomy of your core, master the proper form, discover exciting variations, and design workouts that challenge you at every level. So, get ready to flip your fitness routine upside down and unlock the core of your potential with the incredible inverted row!

Are you ready to join the core revolution? Let's begin!

Chapter 1

# Anatomy of the Core Understanding the Muscles You'll Target

Before diving into the inverted row's magic, let's take a quick anatomy lesson to understand the key players in your core region. While the "six-pack" often steals the spotlight, your core is much more complex and encompasses a deeper level of muscles responsible for stability, power, and movement.

Think of your core as a three-layer cake:

1. Deepest Layer: The local stabilizers are hidden gems, unseen but incredibly important. This layer includes:

- Transversus abdominis (TrA): The deep superstar, providing core rigidity and protecting your spine.
- Multifidus: Runs along your spine, promoting stability and flexibility.
- Diaphragm: Not just for breathing, it also contributes to core tension and intra-abdominal pressure.

2. Middle Layer: The "six-pack" muscles, also known as the global movers, contribute to movement and power. These include:

- Rectus abdominis: The visible "six-pack," responsible for trunk flexion and spinal stability.
- Internal and external obliques: These wrap around your sides, assisting with rotation, bending, and stabilization.

3. Outer Layer: The hip flexors and pelvic floor muscles indirectly connect to your core

and play a crucial role in core stability and function.

How the inverted row activates your core:

The inverted row is unique because it engages all three layers of your core simultaneously:

- Local stabilizers: The TrA fires up to maintain spinal stability as you pull your bodyweight.
- Global movers: The rectus abdominis and obliques work together to control trunk movement and resist rotation.
- Indirectly: The hip flexors and pelvic floor muscles engage to maintain proper alignment and posture throughout the exercise.

By targeting all these muscles, the inverted row builds a comprehensive core that's not just strong, but also functional and resilient.

Next Steps:

- As you progress through the guide, you'll learn how specific variations of the inverted row emphasize different core muscles.
- Visualizing which muscles are working during each exercise can enhance mind-muscle connection and maximize your results.

Remember, building a strong core requires consistent effort and a variety of exercises. The inverted row is a powerful tool in your arsenal, but don't forget to explore other movements to create a well-rounded core training program.

Stay tuned for the next chapter, where we'll master the perfect inverted row form and unlock its full core-activating potential!

Chapter 2

# Master the Basics    Proper Form and Progressions for the Inverted Row

Now that you understand the core muscles the inverted row targets, let's delve into mastering the perfect form. Remember, proper form is crucial for maximizing results and preventing injury. So, ditch the sloppy reps and prepare to nail this exercise like a pro!

Equipment:

- You'll need a sturdy bar, such as a pull-up bar, barbell in a squat rack, or gymnastic rings.
- A padded mat underneath the bar provides extra comfort and protects your lower back.

Setup:

1. Adjust the bar height to challenge you but maintain good form. Ideally, you should be able to hang with your arms extended without touching the floor.
2. Lie on the floor with your face up, directly under the bar.
3. Grab the bar with an overhand grip (palms facing away from you), slightly wider than shoulder-width apart.
4. Engage your core by pulling your belly button towards your spine and brace your glutes.
5. Extend your legs straight out, heels firmly planted on the floor.

The Pull:

1. Initiate the movement by pulling your elbows towards your hips, not raising your chest directly. Imagine squeezing

your shoulder blades together and rowing the bar towards you.

2. As you pull yourself up, keep your body in a straight line from head to heels. Avoid sagging your hips or arching your back.

3. Pull yourself up until your chest nearly touches the bar. Squeeze your core at the top of the movement.

4. Slowly lower yourself back to the starting position with control, maintaining the straight body line and engaged core.

Common Mistakes:

- Kipping: Avoid using momentum (swinging your legs) to complete the reps. Focus on controlled pulls using your back and core muscles.
- Rounding your back: Maintain a flat back throughout the movement to avoid putting strain on your spine.

- Lifting your hips: Keep your body in a straight line and avoid sagging your hips towards the floor.
- Not engaging your core: Remember, your core is the key! Brace your abs and glutes throughout the entire movement.

Progressions:

- Assisted row: Use a resistance band looped around the bar or another object for support until you can perform full bodyweight rows.
- Elevated feet: Place your feet on a platform or bench to reduce the difficulty.
- Knee raises: Hang from the bar and perform knee raises to build upper body strength before progressing to full rows.

- Negatives: Lower yourself down from the top of the movement with control, even if you can't pull yourself up yet.

Remember: Start with a weight or variation that allows you to maintain good form. As you get stronger, gradually increase the difficulty by using less assistance or higher bar positions.

Next Steps:

- Practice the inverted row with proper form until it becomes second nature.
- Explore different variations in the next chapter to target specific core muscles and challenge yourself further.
- Stay focused on form over quantity, and you'll be amazed at how your core strength and definition improve!

Chapter 3

# Safety First  Injury Prevention and Modifications for All Levels

The inverted row is a fantastic core exercise, but like any exercise, it's crucial to prioritize safety and injury prevention. Before you dive into advanced variations, let's address some key safety tips and modifications to ensure you get the most out of your workouts without compromising your well-being.

Warm-up is key:

- Begin your workout with a dynamic warm-up to prepare your muscles and joints for the upcoming exertion. Include light cardio, arm circles, shoulder rolls, and bodyweight squats.

- Specifically dedicate a few minutes to mobilizing your shoulder joints and warming up your core with light planks and bird-dogs.

Listen to your body:

- Pay attention to any pain or discomfort during the exercise. If you experience pain, stop immediately and consult a healthcare professional before continuing.
- Don't push yourself beyond your limits, especially when trying new variations. Start with lighter weights or easier progressions and gradually increase the difficulty as you get stronger.

Proper form is your shield:

- Always prioritize proper form over heavier weights or faster reps. Incorrect form can lead to muscle strain, joint injuries, and other unwanted consequences.

- Refer back to the "Master the Basics" chapter to ensure you're executing the inverted row with perfect technique.

Modifications for different levels:

Beginner:

- Assisted row: Use a resistance band or assisted pull-up machine to reduce the bodyweight you need to lift.
- Negative reps: Hang from the bar and slowly lower yourself down with control, gradually building upper body strength.
- Knee raises: Hang from the bar and perform knee raises to engage your core and upper body.
- Elevated feet: Place your feet on a platform or bench to make the exercise less challenging.

Intermediate:

- Regular inverted row: Once you've mastered the assisted version, progress to full bodyweight rows.
- Single-leg variations: Hold one leg straight out behind you for an increased core challenge.
- Weighted variations: Add weight with a dip belt or by holding a dumbbell between your feet.

Advanced:

- Archer rows: Pull yourself up with one arm at a time for an intense unilateral challenge.
- Explosive rows: Quickly pull yourself up to the top position for added power development.
- Ring rows: Use gymnastic rings for increased instability and core engagement.

Additional tips:

- Maintain a controlled movement throughout the exercise. Avoid jerky motions or swinging your legs for momentum.
- Keep your core engaged throughout the movement for better stability and reduced risk of injury.
- Don't hold your breath. Exhale as you pull yourself up and inhale as you lower yourself down.
- If you have any pre-existing health conditions or injuries, consult a healthcare professional before starting this exercise.

Remember: Safety is paramount. By following these guidelines and listening to your body, you can ensure the inverted row becomes a valuable tool in your core-strengthening journey without compromising your well-being. Now, go forth and conquer your core workouts with confidence!

# Chapter 4

# Equipment Essentials What You Need and Where to Find It

The beauty of the inverted row is that it requires minimal equipment, making it an accessible exercise for almost anyone. Here's a breakdown of the essentials and where you can find them:

1. Pull-up Bar:

- This is the core piece of equipment for inverted rows. You can find them in various forms:
    - Doorway pull-up bars: These are affordable and easy to install, making them a popular choice for home workouts. Just ensure you choose a bar that fits securely in your doorway frame and can support your body weight.

- Wall-mounted pull-up bars: These offer a more permanent solution and can be mounted at different heights to accommodate different exercises.
- Pull-up bars in gyms and parks: Most gyms and many parks have pull-up bars available for public use.

2. Resistance Bands (Optional):

- If you're a beginner or find bodyweight inverted rows too challenging, resistance bands can provide valuable assistance. Look for bands with different resistance levels to adjust the difficulty as you progress.

3. Dip Belt (Optional):

- For advanced athletes looking to add weight to their inverted rows, a dip belt allows you to attach additional weight plates.

4. Gymnastic Rings (Optional):

- These offer a unique challenge and require more core engagement than traditional bars. However, they're not as readily available and require specific mounting points.

5. Exercise Mat (Optional):

- An exercise mat provides cushioning and comfort, especially if you're performing the inverted row on a hard surface.

Remember: Safety is paramount. Ensure your chosen equipment is sturdy, well-maintained, and can support your body weight safely.

When in doubt, consult a trainer or qualified professional for guidance.

With these essentials, you're all set to embark on your inverted row journey and unlock a stronger, more defined core!

Chapter 5

# Beginner Workouts: Get Started and Build a Strong Foundation

Beginner Workout 1:

- Assisted inverted rows: Use a resistance band or assisted pull-up machine to reduce the bodyweight you need to lift. Start with 3 sets of 8-12 repetitions.

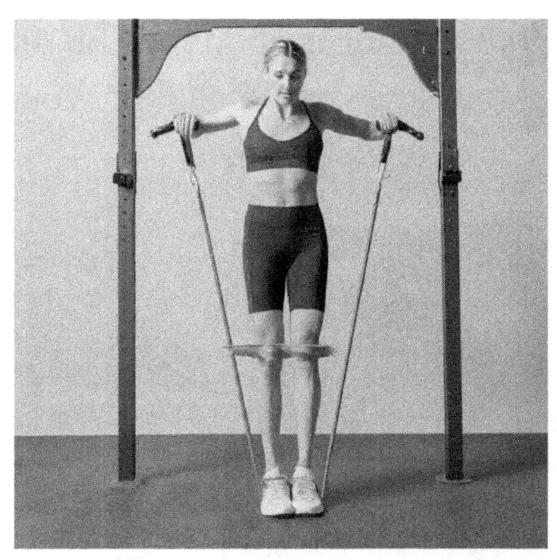

- Plank: Hold a plank position for 30-60 seconds, focusing on engaging your core muscles. Repeat 3 times.

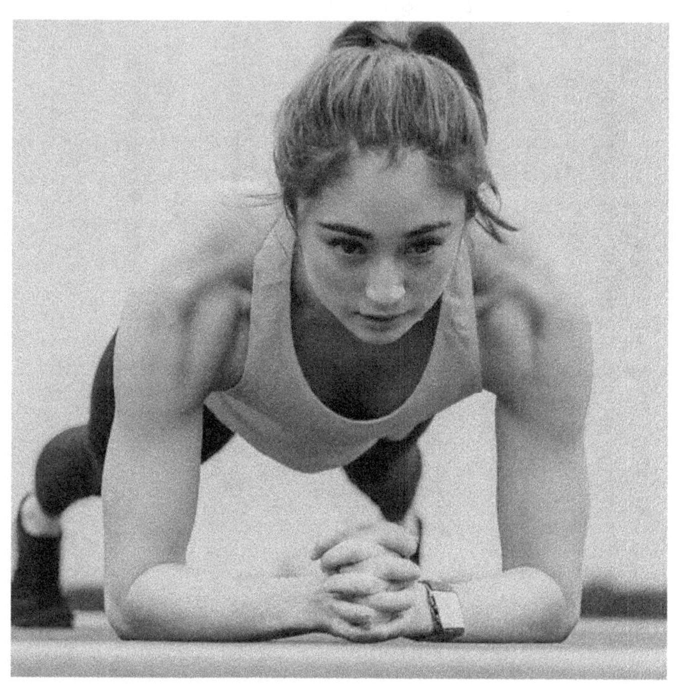

- Bird-dogs: Start on your hands and knees, with your hands shoulder-width apart and your knees hip-width apart. Extend one arm and the opposite leg out straight, keeping your back flat and your core engaged. Hold for a few seconds, then return to starting position. Repeat 10 times on each side.

Beginner Workout 2:

- Negative inverted rows: Hang from the bar and slowly lower yourself down with control. Aim for 3 sets of as many repetitions as you can manage with good form.

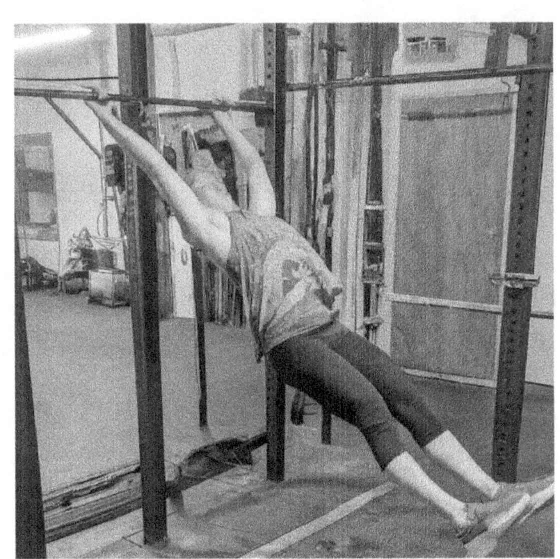

- Side plank: Hold a side plank position on each side for 30-60 seconds, focusing on engaging your core and obliques. Repeat 3 times on each side.

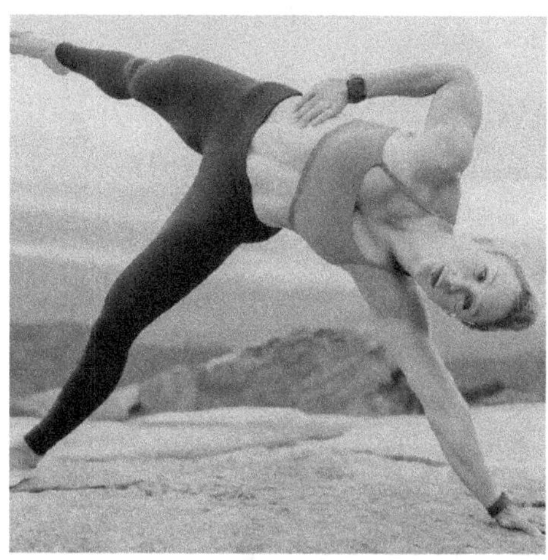

- Dead bugs: Lie on your back with your knees bent and feet flat on the floor. Extend one leg and one arm straight up towards the ceiling, keeping your lower back pressed into the floor. Hold for a few seconds, then return to starting position. Repeat 10 times on each side.

Beginner Workout 3:

- Knee raises: Hang from the bar and bring your knees up towards your chest, keeping your back flat and your core engaged. Lower your legs back down with control. Aim for 3 sets of 10-15 repetitions.

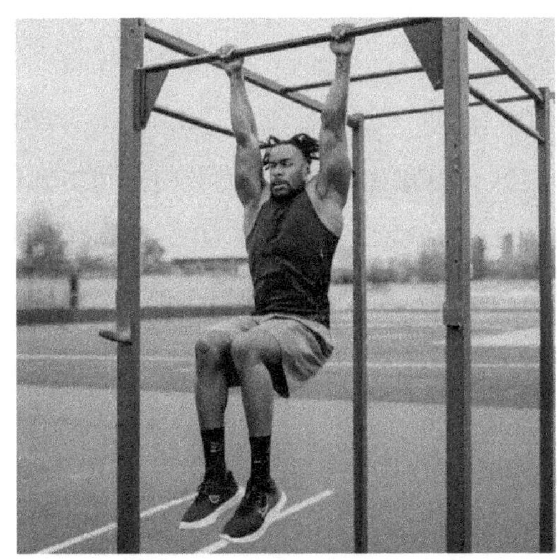

- Russian twists: Sit on the floor with your knees bent and feet flat on the floor. Lean back slightly and twist your torso from side to side, using your core muscles to control the movement. Do 3 sets of 15-20 repetitions.

- Superman: Lie on your stomach with your arms and legs extended out straight. Lift your chest, head, arms, and legs off the ground, squeezing your core muscles. Hold for a few seconds, then lower back down. Repeat 10 times.

These are just a few examples to get you started. As you get stronger, you can progress to more challenging variations of the inverted row and add other exercises to your workouts.

Remember to start with light weights or bodyweight only and gradually increase the difficulty as you get stronger. It's also important to listen to your body and take rest days when needed.

With consistent effort, you'll be on your way to mastering the inverted row and building a strong foundation for your fitness journey!

Here are some additional tips for beginners:

- Focus on proper form over weight. It's more important to do the exercise correctly than to lift a heavy weight.
- Warm up before your workout and cool down afterwards.
- Don't be afraid to ask for help from a trainer or qualified professional.

Chapter 6

# Intermediate Challenges: Take Your Core to the Next Level

Now that you've built a solid foundation with beginner workouts, it's time to challenge your core and take your inverted row skills to the next level! Here are some exciting intermediate variations to push your limits and unlock even more core strength and definition:

Increased Difficulty:

- Full bodyweight inverted rows: Master the basic form using your own bodyweight for an effective core and upper body challenge.

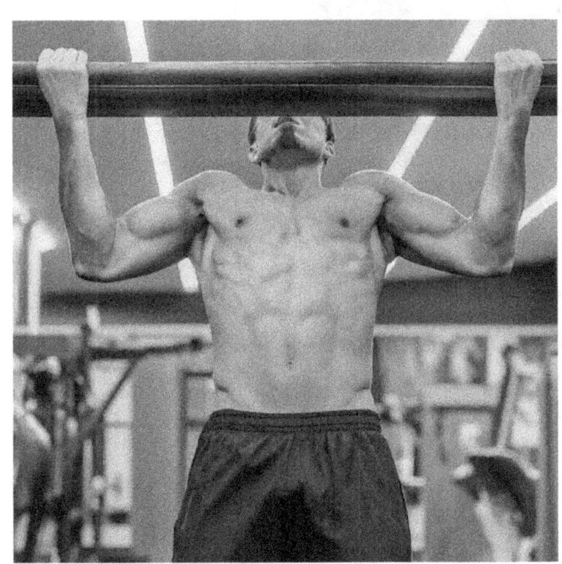

- Single-leg inverted rows: Extend one leg straight out behind you during the pull-up for added core stabilization and unilateral strength development.

- Elevated feet inverted rows: Place your feet on a platform or bench to increase the range of motion and challenge your upper body and core further.

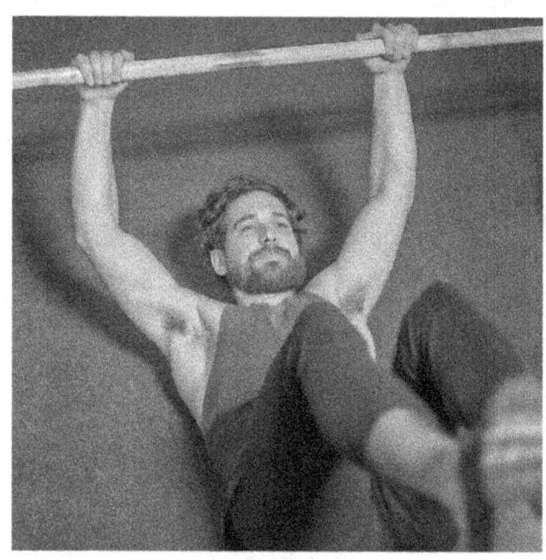

- Weighted inverted rows: Use a dip belt or hold a dumbbell between your feet to add external weight and progressively overload your muscles.

Advanced Variations:

- Archer pull-ups: Pull yourself up with one arm at a time for intense unilateral core engagement and shoulder stability.

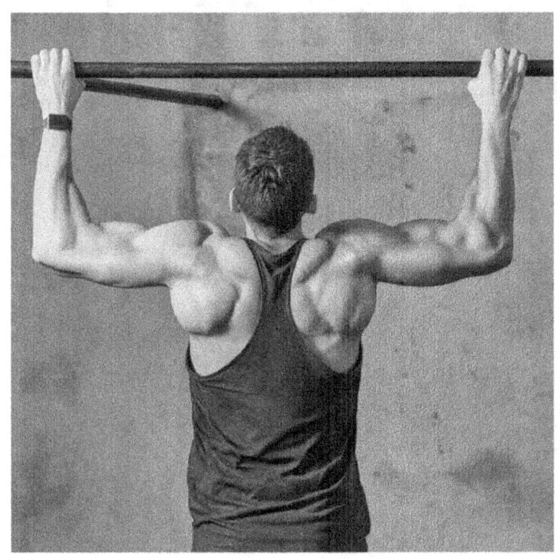

- Explosive inverted rows: Quickly pull yourself up to the top position to develop power and explosiveness in your core and upper body.
- Ring rows: Use gymnastic rings for increased instability and core activation throughout the movement.

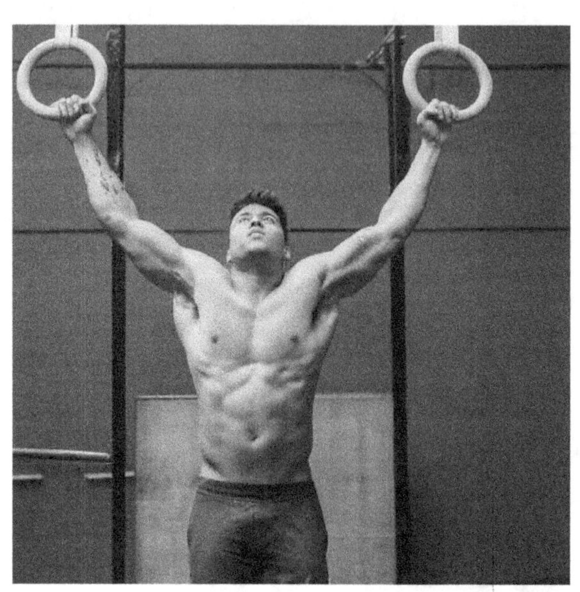

- L-sit holds: Hang from the bar and transition into an L-sit position, holding your legs straight out in front of you for an ultimate core challenge.

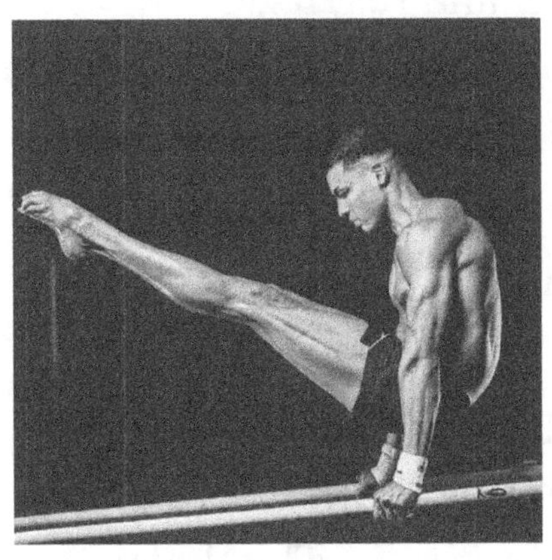

Additional Tips:

- Combine these variations into challenging circuits: Design workouts that combine different inverted row variations with other core exercises like planks, side planks, and Russian twists for a well-rounded core workout.

- Focus on mind-muscle connection: As you perform each variation, visualize your core muscles working and engaging throughout the movement for better activation and results.
- Maintain proper form: Don't sacrifice form for heavier weights or faster reps. Prioritize controlled movements and focus on technique to prevent injury and maximize effectiveness.
- Track your progress: Monitor your performance by recording sets, reps, weights, and rest times. This helps you track your progress and adjust your workouts accordingly.

Remember: Consistency is key! Regularly incorporating these intermediate challenges into your workouts will lead to significant improvements in your core strength, stability, and definition. Embrace the challenge, push your limits safely, and witness your core transform to the next level!

Chapter 7

# Advanced Variations: Push Your Limits and Maximize Results

Ready to truly supercharge your core with the inverted row? Buckle up, because these advanced variations will challenge even the most seasoned athletes. But remember, safety and proper form are paramount. Master the basics and consult a qualified trainer before attempting these intense exercises.

Explosive Power:

Jumping Inverted Rows: Explode off the bar at the top of the pull-up, momentarily defying gravity and maximizing power output.

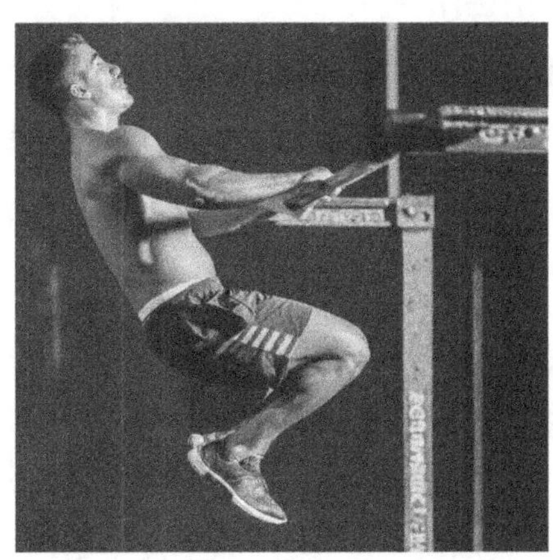

- Plyometric Knees-to-Chest: Add a jump to your knees-to-chest pull-ups, boosting core and leg explosiveness.
- Medicine Ball Slams: After each regular inverted row, slam a medicine ball on the ground, combining upper body pulling power with core stability.

Advanced Strength:

- Weighted Muscle-Ups: Add weight using a dip belt or vest to challenge your entire upper body and core in this dynamic movement.
- Weighted One-Arm Inverted Rows: Master regular one-arm rows and gradually add weight for incredible unilateral strength and core control.
- Dragon Flag: Progress from front levers to the advanced dragon flag, holding your body parallel to the ground with only your core and shoulders engaged.

Unilateral Mastery:

- Alternating Single-Arm Rows: Continuously alternate arms during the pull-up phase, maintaining core stability and challenging shoulder stability.

- Windmill Rows: Perform single-arm rows while walking laterally, adding core engagement and coordination.
- Side Plank Row: Hold a side plank position and perform single-arm rows, integrating core and shoulder stability in a unique way.

Advanced Circuit Example:

- 3 sets of:
    - 5 Jumping Inverted Rows
    - 8 Weighted Muscle-Ups
    - 10 Alternating Single-Arm Rows (each side)
    - 30-second Dragon Flag Hold
    - Rest 3 minutes between sets

Remember:

- Advanced doesn't mean reckless: Only attempt these variations with proper form and adequate conditioning.
- Start light and progress gradually: Increase weight, reps, or difficulty over time to avoid injury.
- Prioritize safety: Wear appropriate shoes and attire, and train in a safe environment.
- Listen to your body: Take rest days and consult a healthcare professional if you experience any pain or discomfort.

By incorporating these advanced variations and prioritizing safety, you can unlock the full potential of the inverted row and achieve a powerful, defined core that will impress. Remember, consistent effort and smart training are key to achieving your fitness goals. Push your limits, but always prioritize proper form and listen to your body. Good luck!

Chapter 8

# Core Circuits: Combine the Inverted Row with Other Bodyweight Exercises

The inverted row reigns supreme as a core-strengthening exercise, but its magic doesn't stop there! By incorporating it into bodyweight circuits, you can unlock a whole new level of functional fitness, sculpting a strong, defined core while challenging your entire body.

Why circuit training?

Circuit training combines multiple exercises with minimal rest periods, creating a dynamic and efficient workout that keeps your heart rate up and your core constantly engaged. This not only blasts calories but also builds endurance, coordination, and agility – all essential for a well-rounded fitness routine.

The Inverted Row as Your Anchor:

Think of the inverted row as the anchor of your circuit. Each rep fires up your core, while its pulling motion complements various bodyweight exercises, creating a cohesive and challenging flow. Here are some circuit ideas to get you started:

Circuit 1: Metabolic Meltdown

- Inverted Rows (3 sets of 8 reps)
- Jumping Squats (3 sets of 12 reps)
- Push-ups (3 sets of max reps)
- Mountain Climbers (3 sets of 30 seconds)
- Rest: 30 seconds between exercises, 1 minute between circuits

Circuit 2: Upper Body Blitz

- Inverted Rows (3 sets of 10 reps)
- Dips on a chair (3 sets of max reps)

- Renegade Rows (3 sets of 8 reps per side)
- Plank with Shoulder Taps (3 sets of 30 seconds)
- Rest: 30 seconds between exercises, 1 minute between circuits

Circuit 3: Agility Challenge

- Inverted Rows with Leg Raise (3 sets of 6 reps)
- Burpees (3 sets of 8 reps)
- Lateral Shuffles (3 sets of 30 seconds each side)
- High Knees (3 sets of 30 seconds)
- Rest: 30 seconds between exercises, 1 minute between circuits

Remember:

- Modify exercises based on your fitness level. Opt for knee push-ups or wall dips if needed.

- Listen to your body and take rest days when needed.
- Gradually increase the difficulty by adding more reps, sets, or reducing rest time.
- Most importantly, have fun and challenge yourself!

Bonus Tip: Add a medicine ball or resistance band to any of these circuits for an extra challenge.

Embrace the Circuit:

These are just a few examples to spark your creativity. Design your own circuits, experiment with different exercises, and most importantly, have fun! Remember, the inverted row is your gateway to a stronger, more versatile core, and bodyweight circuits are your key to unlocking its full potential. So, get moving, get creative, and experience the transformative power of the circuit!

Chapter 9

# Training Tips: Optimize Your Workouts for Faster Core Progress with the Inverted Row

So you're ready to maximize your gains and accelerate your core development with the inverted row? Excellent! Here are some key training tips to help you optimize your workouts and witness faster progress:

Intensity Matters:

- Progressive overload: Gradually increase the difficulty of your workouts over time. This could involve adding weight, increasing reps/sets, shortening rest periods, or trying more challenging variations.

- Challenge yourself: Don't get stuck in a rut! Step outside your comfort zone and push your limits safely to stimulate muscle growth and adaptation.
- Track your progress: Monitor your reps, sets, weights, and rest times to track your progress and adjust your workouts accordingly.

Mind-Muscle Connection:

- Focus on quality: Don't just go through the motions. Concentrate on engaging your core muscles throughout each movement. Visualize them working and contracting for better activation.
- Slow and controlled: Avoid rapid, jerky movements. Perform each pull-up with control and focus on the full range of motion.
- Mind-muscle connection exercises: Include targeted core exercises like planks, side planks, and bird-dogs

alongside your inverted rows for overall core development.

Recovery and Consistency:

- Schedule rest days: Allow your muscles time to recover and rebuild. Aim for at least 1-2 rest days per week between inverted row workouts.
- Fuel your body: Eat a healthy diet rich in protein and complex carbohydrates to provide your muscles with the nutrients they need to grow and repair.
- Stay hydrated: Drink plenty of water throughout the day to stay hydrated and support muscle function.
- Sleep is essential: Aim for 7-8 hours of quality sleep each night for optimal recovery and hormone balance.

Additional Tips:

- Warm-up and cool down: Prepare your muscles with a dynamic warm-up and cool down with static stretches to prevent injury.
- Variety is key: Don't stick to the same routine every day. Mix up your workout exercises and variations to keep your core engaged and challenged.
- Seek guidance: Consider working with a certified personal trainer for personalized workout plans and technique feedback.
- Listen to your body: Take rest days if needed and stop any exercise that causes pain.

Remember, consistency is key. Stick to your training program, incorporate these tips, and witness your core transform with the amazing inverted row!

Disclaimer: This information is for educational purposes only and should not substitute for professional medical advice. Always consult a healthcare professional before starting any new exercise program.

Chapter 10

# Building Functional Strength: How the Inverted Row Benefits Your Entire Body

The inverted row isn't just a core powerhouse; it's a functional strength machine that benefits your entire body in surprising ways. Beyond sculpted abs, here's how this exercise:

Enhances Upper Body Strength and Power:

- Targets multiple muscle groups: Pull-ups primarily activate your back (lats, traps), but the inverted row engages additional muscles like biceps, shoulders (delts), and forearms for a well-rounded upper body workout.

- Improves pulling strength: Pulling movements are crucial for everyday activities like opening doors, climbing stairs, and carrying groceries. The inverted row strengthens these muscles for improved daily function and athletic performance.
- Builds back stability: A strong back supports good posture and protects your spine from injury. The inverted row strengthens your back muscles, promoting better posture and reducing risk of back pain.

Boosts Core Stability and Function:

- Engages your entire core: Unlike crunches that target specific abdominal muscles, the inverted row activates your entire core, including the deep core muscles essential for stability and injury prevention.

- Develops anti-rotational strength: The inverted row forces your core to resist rotational forces, mimicking real-life movements and improving core stability for various activities.
- Strengthens your pelvic floor: Indirectly, the inverted row engages your pelvic floor muscles, crucial for bladder and bowel control, sexual function, and overall core health.

Improves Shoulder Health and Mobility:

- Full range of motion: The inverted row utilizes a full range of shoulder motion, promoting flexibility and stability in your shoulder joints.
- Prevents shoulder imbalances: Many exercises focus on pushing movements (push-ups), neglecting important pulling movements. The inverted row balances your shoulder development and prevents muscle imbalances.

- Reduces risk of shoulder injuries: Strong and mobile shoulders are less prone to injuries during daily activities and exercise.

Additional Benefits:

- Increased grip strength: Holding onto the bar strengthens your forearms and grip, improving your performance in other exercises and daily tasks.
- Enhanced athletic performance: The inverted row improves various aspects of athletic performance, including power, strength, and stability.
- Weight management: Building muscle mass can boost your metabolism and aid in weight management efforts.

Remember, the inverted row is a versatile exercise that offers tremendous benefits beyond just core strength. So, incorporate it into your workout routine and experience the positive impact it has on your entire body!

Disclaimer: This information is for educational purposes only and should not substitute for professional medical advice. Always consult a healthcare professional before starting any new exercise program.

Chapter 11

# Nutrition for Core Activation: Fueling Your Workouts for Success

You're on the right track to maximizing your core workouts with the inverted row! But remember, nutrition plays a crucial role in fueling your body and optimizing your results. Here's how to adjust your diet to support core activation and performance:

Macronutrients Matter:

- Protein: The building block of muscle! Aim for 0.8-1 gram of protein per pound of body weight daily to support muscle growth and repair, especially after intense workouts. Lean protein sources like chicken, fish, tofu, and beans are excellent choices.

- Carbohydrates: Provide energy for your workouts. Choose complex carbs like whole grains, fruits, and vegetables for sustained energy and avoid sugary processed options that can cause crashes.
- Healthy Fats: Don't fear fats! They contribute to hormone production, cell function, and satiety. Include healthy fats from sources like nuts, seeds, avocados, and olive oil in your diet.

Micronutrients are Mighty:

- Hydration: Crucial for muscle function and performance. Aim for at least 8 glasses of water daily, and adjust based on your activity level and climate.
- Electrolytes: Minerals like sodium, potassium, and magnesium help maintain fluid balance and muscle

function. Replenish electrolytes lost through sweat with sports drinks or natural sources like coconut water.

- Vitamins and Minerals: Support overall health and energy levels. Consume a variety of fruits, vegetables, and whole grains to ensure you're getting essential vitamins and minerals.

Pre- and Post-Workout Nutrition:

- Pre-workout: Aim for a small, easily digestible snack rich in carbs and protein 30-60 minutes before your workout. This provides energy and helps prevent muscle breakdown.
- Post-workout: Replenish glycogen stores and support muscle recovery with a meal or snack containing protein and carbs within 30-60 minutes after your workout.

Additional Tips:

- Listen to your body: Adjust your calorie intake and food choices based on your individual needs and activity level.
- Consult a nutritionist: Consider seeking guidance from a registered dietitian or nutritionist for personalized dietary advice.
- Stay hydrated: Drink water throughout the day, especially before, during, and after your workouts.
- Focus on whole foods: Prioritize unprocessed, whole foods over processed options for optimal nutrition.

Remember, nutrition is a journey, not a destination. Experiment with different foods and find what works best for your body and training goals. By fueling your body with the right nutrients, you'll unlock the full potential of your core workouts and achieve even better results!

Disclaimer: This information is for educational purposes only and should not substitute for professional medical advice. Always consult a healthcare professional or registered dietitian before making significant changes to your diet.

Chapter 12

# Staying Motivated: Tips and Strategies to Maintain Your Fitness Journey

Staying motivated on your fitness journey can be challenging, especially when life gets busy or routines change. But fear not, there are plenty of tips and strategies you can use to keep the fire burning and your core workouts consistent with the inverted row!

Internal Motivation:

- Connect to your WHY: Remind yourself why you started this journey in the first place. Is it for improved health, stronger core, more energy, or a specific event? Visualize your goals and how achieving them will positively impact your life.

- Celebrate small wins: Track your progress, even small achievements, and acknowledge your effort. Reward yourself for reaching milestones to reinforce positive behaviors.
- Find the joy in movement: Make exercise enjoyable! Explore different workout styles, find activities you genuinely enjoy, and listen to music that pumps you up.
- Challenge yourself: Step outside your comfort zone and try new variations of the inverted row or other exercises. Keep things interesting to avoid boredom.

External Motivation:

- Find a workout buddy: Partnering up for workouts can increase accountability and make exercise more social and fun.

- Join a fitness class: Group classes provide a structured environment, community support, and motivation from the instructor and other participants.

- Hire a personal trainer: A personal trainer can create a personalized program, offer guidance, and provide motivation through encouragement and feedback.

- Track your progress: Use fitness trackers, apps, or journals to log your workouts, reps, and progress. Seeing your hard work quantified can be incredibly motivating.

- Share your journey: Tell your friends and family about your goals and progress. Having their support and encouragement can make a big difference.

- Reward yourself: Set up a reward system for achieving certain milestones or sticking to your workout routine. This could be anything from a new workout outfit to a relaxing massage.

Additional Tips:

- Focus on progress, not perfection: Don't get discouraged by setbacks. Everyone has them! Just get back on track and keep moving forward.
- Plan your workouts: Schedule your workouts in advance and treat them like important appointments. This will help you stay committed.
- Make it convenient: Keep your workout clothes and equipment readily available, and choose workout times that fit your schedule.
- Listen to your body: Take rest days when needed and don't push yourself too hard. Overtraining can lead to injuries and burnout.

- Find inspiration: Read fitness blogs, watch motivational videos, or follow inspiring fitness figures on social media.

Remember, motivation is a journey, not a destination. There will be ups and downs, but by incorporating these tips and strategies, you can stay committed to your core workouts with the inverted row and achieve your fitness goals!

Disclaimer: This information is for educational purposes only and should not substitute for professional medical advice. Always consult a healthcare professional before starting any new exercise program.

Chapter 13

# Common Mistakes and How to Avoid Them

Even the most dedicated exercisers can make mistakes, and the inverted row is no exception. Here are some common mistakes to watch out for and how to avoid them:

Form Flaws:

- Hunching your back: Keep your core engaged and back straight throughout the movement. Imagine pulling yourself up with your chest, not just your arms.
- Letting your hips sag: Engage your glutes and core to maintain a straight line from your head to your heels.

Think of holding a plank position while pulling yourself up.

- Swinging your legs: Use controlled movements and focus on pulling yourself up with your upper body strength. Avoid using momentum from your legs.
- Gripping too wide or narrow: A shoulder-width grip is generally optimal. Experiment to find what feels most comfortable and allows for full range of motion.
- Not fully extending your arms at the bottom: Lower yourself until your arms are fully extended with a slight lean back. This ensures you're working the full range of motion.

Other Mistakes:

- Starting too heavy: Begin with bodyweight or light weights and gradually increase the difficulty as you get stronger. Improper form with heavy weights can lead to injury.

- Neglecting your warm-up and cool-down: Prepare your muscles with a dynamic warm-up and cool down with static stretches to prevent injury.
- Overtraining: Listen to your body and take rest days when needed. Pushing yourself too hard can lead to fatigue, decreased performance, and increased risk of injury.
- Not prioritizing recovery: Ensure adequate sleep, hydration, and a nutritious diet to support muscle recovery and overall health.
- Comparing yourself to others: Everyone progresses at their own pace. Focus on your own journey and celebrate your personal achievements.

Additional Tips:

- Pay attention to your body: Stop if you experience any pain or discomfort. It's better to adjust your form or take a break than risk injury.
- Record yourself: Videoing yourself performing the exercise can help you identify and correct any form issues.
- Seek guidance: Consider working with a qualified trainer for personalized instruction and feedback on your technique.

Remember, consistency and proper form are key to maximizing your results and avoiding injury. By being mindful of these common mistakes and incorporating the tips provided, you can ensure your inverted row journey is safe, effective, and leads you towards a stronger, more defined core!

Chapter 14

# Frequently Asked Questions about the Inverted Row:

1. Can I do inverted rows if I can't do pull-ups?

Absolutely! Inverted rows are a great way to build the strength needed for pull-ups. Start with bodyweight or assisted inverted rows using resistance bands or a pull-up machine, and gradually progress to full pull-ups as you get stronger.

2. How often should I do inverted rows?

Aim for 2-3 sets of 8-12 repetitions, 2-3 times per week. Allow your muscles rest and recovery time between workouts.

3. What are some good variations of the inverted row?

There are many variations to challenge yourself as you progress. Here are a few:

- Elevated feet inverted rows: Place your feet on a platform or bench for a greater range of motion.
- Weighted inverted rows: Add weight using a dip belt or dumbbell held between your feet.
- Single-leg inverted rows: Extend one leg straight out behind you for added core engagement.
- Archer pull-ups: Alternate pulling yourself up with one arm at a time.

4. Are inverted rows good for my back?

Yes, inverted rows are a fantastic exercise for strengthening your back muscles, particularly your lats, traps, and rhomboids. They also engage your core and shoulders for a well-rounded upper body workout.

5. Can I do inverted rows at home?

Definitely! You can use a doorway pull-up bar, wall-mounted pull-up bar, or even a sturdy table or chair with a secure grip.

6. What are some common mistakes to avoid when doing inverted rows?

- Hunching your back. Maintain a straight back and core engagement throughout the movement.
- Swinging your legs. Focus on pulling yourself up with your upper body strength, not momentum.
- Using too heavy weight. Start with bodyweight or light weights and progress gradually.
- Neglecting your warm-up and cool-down.

7. Where can I find more information about inverted rows?

There are many online resources and fitness professionals who can offer guidance and tips for performing inverted rows. Additionally, consider consulting a certified personal trainer for personalized instruction and feedback on your technique.

Remember: Listen to your body, prioritize proper form, and be consistent in your workouts for optimal results with the inverted row!

**Bonus**

Chapter 15

# Sample Workout Logs and Tracking Sheets for Inverted Rows

Here is the link for the workout logs and tracking sheets
https://docs.google.com/spreadsheets/d/1K1C
NmBPour3ceHduGzJnx2Z3UN0JlDhwIncjks
0GKN4/edit?usp=drivesdk
Additional Tips:

- You can create your own logs and sheets using simple tools like paper or spreadsheets, or utilize dedicated fitness apps for more features.
- Adapt the logs and sheets to your specific goals and preferences.

- Be consistent with your tracking to monitor your progress and make adjustments as needed.
- Use notes to record any observations, feelings, or adjustments made during your workouts.

Remember, tracking your progress is a valuable tool for staying motivated and achieving your fitness goals with the inverted row!

Chapter 15

# In-Depth Anatomy Diagrams and Illustrations

Sure, here are some in-depth anatomy diagrams and illustrations of the muscles involved in the inverted row exercise:

- The muscles of the back: The inverted row primarily targets the latissimus dorsi (lats), which are the large muscles on the sides of your back. They are responsible for pulling your arms downward and backward. The rhomboids and trapezius muscles also play a role in this movement.
- The muscles of the core: The inverted row also engages your core muscles, including the rectus abdominis, obliques, and transverse abdominis.

These muscles help to stabilize your spine and pelvis during the movement.

- The muscles of the arms: The biceps brachii and brachialis muscles in your upper arms help to bend your elbows and pull your body up during the inverted row. The forearms muscles are also engaged in gripping the bar.

By understanding the muscles involved in the inverted row, you can focus on engaging them properly during the exercise to maximize your results.

Here are some additional tips for performing the inverted row with proper form:

- Keep your back straight and core engaged throughout the movement.
- Pull yourself up towards your chest, not just your chin.
- Lower yourself down slowly and with control.

- Don't use momentum to swing your body up.
- Choose a weight that is challenging but allows you to maintain good form.

With proper form and consistent practice, the inverted row can be a great exercise for strengthening your back, core, and arms.

# Conclusion

Mastering the Inverted Row - Your Gateway to a Stronger, Empowered You

As you reach the final page of this journey, we hope you've gained a deep understanding and appreciation for the transformative power of the inverted row. This simple yet potent exercise is more than just a core-sculpting tool; it's a gateway to a stronger, more empowered you.

Throughout this book, you've explored the inverted row's anatomy, biomechanics, and its impact on various aspects of your physical health. You've learned proper form, mastered different variations, and unlocked tips and strategies to optimize your workouts.

Remember, the true power of the inverted row lies not only in the physical gains, but also in the journey itself. The dedication, discipline, and self-belief you cultivate through consistent practice will spill over into other areas of your life, empowering you to tackle challenges and achieve your goals.

Here are some key takeaways to carry with you:

- The inverted row is a versatile exercise that benefits your entire body, from core strength and upper body power to improved posture and mobility.
- Mastering proper form is crucial to maximize effectiveness and prevent injury.
- Consistency is key. Embrace the journey, celebrate small wins, and trust the process.
- Challenge yourself with progressions and variations to keep things interesting and push your limits.
- Listen to your body, prioritize recovery, and don't be afraid to seek guidance.

As you move forward, let the inverted row serve as a symbol of your dedication and achievement. Remember the strength you've built, the challenges you've overcome, and the confidence you've gained. Go forth and conquer your goals, both in the gym and beyond!

This is not just the end of a book, but the beginning of a stronger, more empowered you. Keep pulling, keep challenging yourself, and remember, the power lies within.

# Request for a review

A heartfelt plea for honest feedback: Help elevate my book and others discover its power!

As you reach the final page of my book, a wave of emotions washes over me – gratitude for your time, pride in the journey, and a touch of trepidation. You see, a writer's work thrives on connection, and your honest feedback is the lifeblood that nourishes growth and fuels future endeavors.

This book may have resonated with you, challenged you, or even sparked unexpected conversations within yourself. That's exactly what I hoped for! But my journey doesn't end here. I strive to reach others who might benefit from this knowledge, and your valuable review holds the key to unlocking that door.

Here's how your review can make a difference:

- Help potential readers discover the book: Your genuine opinion and insights can attract others who might find value in its pages.
- Shape my writing journey: Every piece of feedback, positive or constructive, helps me refine my craft and create even better content in the future.
- Build a community of like-minded individuals: Your review can spark conversations and connect you with others who share your interest in the book's themes.

Remember, there's no pressure to write a lengthy critique. Even a few sentences about what resonated with you or areas you found particularly helpful can make a world of difference.

Thank you from the bottom of my heart for considering my request. Your support means more than words can express.

Together, let's build a community around this book and empower others to discover the transformational power of the inverted row!

Warmly,

Helen Talbott

P.S. If you have any specific questions or thoughts you'd like to share directly with me, feel free to reach out! I'm always happy to connect with my readers.